UNLOCK DYSLEXIA:
A COMPREHENSIVE WORKBOOK

Unleash Your Potential.

Jared J. Makheja

The Elevator Project LLC
1390 Chain Bridge Road, Suite 170
McLean, Virginia 22101

www.unlockdyslexia.com

Ordering Information:

Quantity sales. Special discounts are available on quantity purchases by corporations, associations, and others. For details, contact the publisher at the address above.

Printed in the United States of America
First Edition
ISBN: 978-1-48358-097-5

Contents

Contents (contd.)

Dedication

This book is dedicated to all of the persistent dyslexics in the world, who never give up and continue to try to learn everyday. Remember to never surrender because difficult roads lead to beautiful destinations.

Foreword:

Jared Makheja's workbook provides guidance for dyslexics, teachers, doctors, and dyslexia advocates through extensive knowledge and background regarding dyslexia. It also provides cognitive exercises to help dyslexics develop the skills they might be lacking. No person truly understands what it is like to be dyslexic, unless dyslexia has, in some way, touched their lives. Even then, most people affected by dyslexia do not have background knowledge on dyslexia nor do they know exactly what to do to help. As a doctor, I have spent years studying various learning disabilities, and there is a lot of information and background needed in order to have a good understanding of dyslexia. However, upon reading *Unlock Dyslexia: A Comprehensive Workbook*, understanding dyslexia and therapeutic methods for dyslexics became clear as the majority of the information surrounding the learning disability is covered in a comprehensive manner.

I am sure using some of this workbook's exercises will yield tremendous positive rewards with improved fluency in reading and increased comprehension and attitude towards developing reading skills. Jared Makheja's dedication to changing outcomes, not only in the world of learning disabilities but also in neurology and cognitive physiology, shines through this book.

- Darshan Kumar, M.D.

Renu Health Clinic

Preface

A study in 2014 by the National Center for Learning Disabilities stated the prevalence of those with learning disabilities living in poverty doubles the prevalence of those with learning disabilities not living in poverty. After reading this horrific fact, I began an organization, The Elevator Project Special Needs Program, which is dedicated to lifting those with learning disabilities out of poverty through individualized training of vocational and interpersonal skills, giving the individual the skills to acquire a full-time job and lift them and their families out of poverty. Through the organization, I have noticed that in addition to a customized training program, individuals with learning disabilities also need neuro-strengthening programs, where not only are they learning their specific trade, they are fully developing the learning skills they may be lacking. Furthermore, I noticed that loved ones and friends of those impacted by learning disabilities want to help. However, they lack the knowledge about the learning disability and do not know what to do to assist their friend or loved one.

As a result, I have developed many detailed, comprehensive guides in *Unlock Dyslexia: A Comprehensive Workbook* to help the families and friends of those with learning disabilities. *Unlock Dyslexia* begins with a comprehensive overview of dyslexia, how people are affected by it, and what are some learning aids to help those with dyslexia. Then, the workbook goes into three major impacted areas of dyslexia: the sense of sight, hearing, and spatial. For each of these impacted areas, there is a lesson on how to improve a) recognition, b) memory, and c) sequencing, along with body perception and spatial orientation. Under each impacted area, the workbook explains the science and the effect on dyslexics followed by three levels of curative exercises which increase in the level of difficulty as it builds the neuropathways in the dyslexic participant.

Dyslexia: An Overview

What is dyslexia?

Dyslexia is a learning disability that affects the structural alignment of the brain. A learning disability is a disorder in the mental processes used for qualitative or quantitative reasoning. The disorder occurs in people of normal or above-normal intelligence. In addition, some challenges that arise because of dyslexia are not the result of eye, ear, or motivational difficulties, rather the brain is not processing or perceiving the information and data that the sensory receptors are receiving. In addition, it is not the result of emotional disturbance. When you have dyslexia, you are challenged when facing the obstacle of comprehending written words. Therefore you also have difficulty writing. Those with dyslexic brains do not recognize that words are made up of small units of sound, known as phonemes. Dyslexia can be diagnosed by taking a basic diagnostic cognitive test. This test both informs one of whether he/she has dyslexia or not, but also to what degree of dyslexia he/she has.

How many people are affected by dyslexia?

Dyslexia affects many people. 15% of the population is affected by a significant difficulty like learning to read. 22% of the dyslexic population live in poverty. However, 12% of all adults living below the poverty line has dyslexia. Dyslexia most commonly affects men as 80% of dyslexics are men.

Why do people have dyslexia?

Many do not know why people have dyslexia; however, scientists and neurologists say dyslexia is rooted in the left side of the brain thus making the under compensation of white and gray matter in the left parietotemporal lobe in the left hemisphere of the brain the makeup of a dyslexic brain. It is very common for a learning disability to be hereditary, especially dyslexia, the most common learning disability. Many studies have shown that dyslexia is hereditary, but not a dominant gene and is shown over many genes. Therefore, if a parent has dyslexia, it does not necessarily mean the child will most definitely have dyslexia. However, the chances are higher. Scientists have wondered for many years how to discover dyslexia at a very early age. Recent studies have shown there is a blood test to discover if you have a learning disability. The blood of the parents and the child must be taken and examined, especially the DNA of the parents. This new development is helpful because if the learning disability is discovered early in the child's life, the parents are able to get specialized training and place the child in a special development program. Dyslexia is usually diagnosed after age six because it is acceptable if you cannot read or write before age six, but with this blood test, one can know if you have a learning disability much earlier. All children are born not knowing how to read, and therefore must be taught. Children are not usually taught to fluently read, and are not expected to read until they are approximately six years old, therefore, if you know at the child's birth that the child is dyslexic, then appropriate teaching actions can be completed so the child's brain can develop at a regular pace of learning, but in a different way. Otherwise, if nobody knew the child was dyslexic, then at the age of six or seven, the child would have lost many critical years of their life trying to do an action that could not be done otherwise. Then, the child would have to catch up to the "regular" learning pace and make the critical years of the child's life stressful and difficult.

THE HUMAN BRAIN

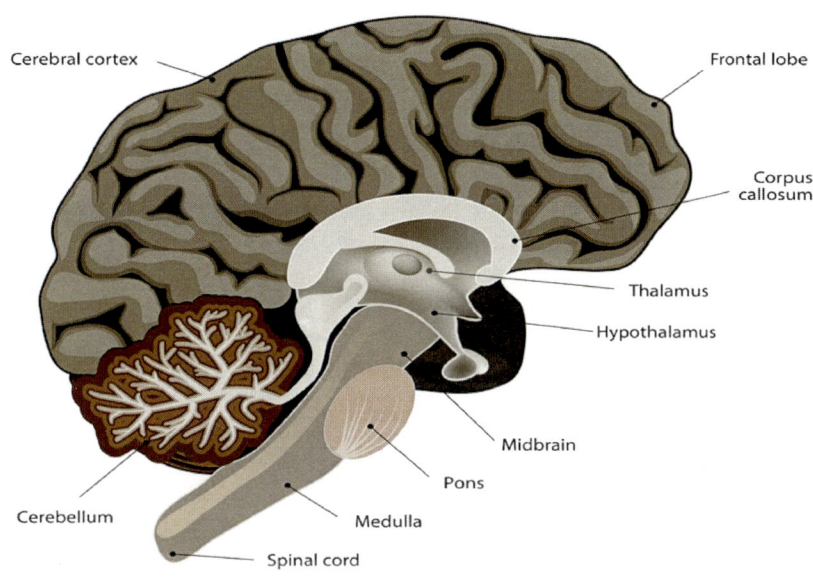

What learning aids help those with dyslexia?

There are many helpful tools that teach those with dyslexia in a style that is more comprehensive for them. For example, text-to-speech pens are helpful to those with dyslexia because they can understand the phonemes or sounds of the words they highlight with their pens and they understand how the sounds look therefore helping them to write. This is a form of learning called auditory processing which is when someone hears something, they understand it more than when they do it or look at it. Another example of learning is called kinesthetic learning which is when someone does the action in order to understand it. For example, instead of sitting in a classroom being taught to fix an electrical problem, they would do it or watch someone do it. Kinesthetic learning is very hands-on and makes the person understand what it is they are doing.

Another very important tool is the type of specific exercises provided in this workbook which strengthen a dyslexic's sense of sight, hearing and spatial perception which is covered in great detail on the following sections of the book.

Section I: The Sense of Sight

Importance

Vision is the process of perceiving information from what is seen. The process of vision is complex and developed from using a multitude of different components. Approximately 85% of our learning, perceptions, and cognitions are a result of vision, therefore making the sense of sight a human's most valuable sense. The process of vision can be broken down into three major categories: visual acuity, visual perception, and visual motor abilities. Dyslexics often have challenges that relate to visual perception.

Visual Acuity

Visual acuity is the clarity of one's sight. It is often measured using the Snellen chart. Visual acuity is often blurred in different refractive conditions, like nearsightedness, farsightedness, or age-related loss of focusing. Visual acuity is noted numerically, for example, 20/20, 20/40, etc. Visual acuity covers the entire visual field, which is the complete peripheral and central range of vision.

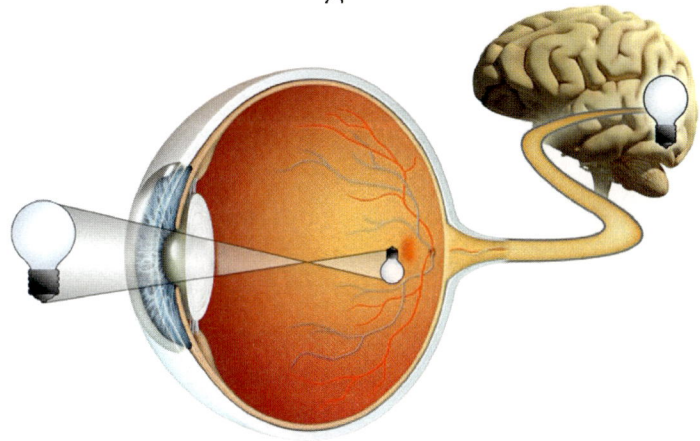

Visual Perception

Visual perception is the ability to integrate the information and data seen to the other senses to have coordination, spatial recognition, and in order to do cognitive functions.

Visual Motor Functions

Visual motor functions refer to the movement of the eyes and the rapid focusing and aiming of the eyes to retain the information. Visual motor functions include the ability to focus on an object, sustain that focus, accurately use the eyes to track or follow a moving object, use the eyes to quickly and precisely scan and look at different objects, and aim the eyes to look at a specific object. In addition, visual motor functions include depth perception and the integration of convergence and accommodation of the eyes.

Visual Exercises

The following three lessons and worksheets focus on recognition, memory, and sequencing respectively and how they impact one's reading skills and function with regards to brain activity. After each lesson there is a series of three exercise that increase in difficulty strengthen a dyslexic brain in that specific area.

Section I Lesson 1: Visual Recognition

Overview

Visual recognition is the ability to perceive letters quickly and accurately. Visual recognition is a major component in order to fluently and efficiently read, as reading requires phoneme-grapheme correspondence. Phoneme-grapheme correspondence is one of the many underlying capacities needed for reading and involves the integration of sounds (phonemes) and letters (graphemes). Normally, young children develop the ability to visually recognize letters and words. Therefore, as the child's brain networks mature, so they are able to read fluently as they get older. This is why the human brain is not "wired" to know how to read.

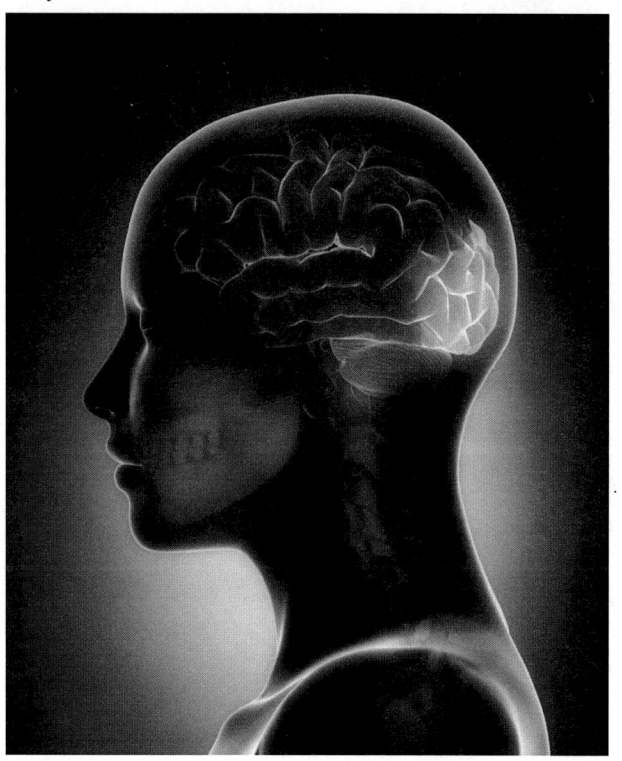

The Science: The Brain and Reading

The human brain is divided into many different areas. The visual word formation area of the brain, where the visual recognition ability is located, is at the base of left hemisphere. The base of the left hemisphere is the occipital lobe and controls the majority of the visual abilities of the body. The specific area of the brain that the visual recognition ability is located in is often termed the "letter-box". The "letter-box" area shows stronger stimulation to written words and letters rather than any other type of visual stimulus, like places, faces, or objects. For many, the "letter-box" area is located between the areas of the base of the left hemisphere that are stimulated due to places and objects.

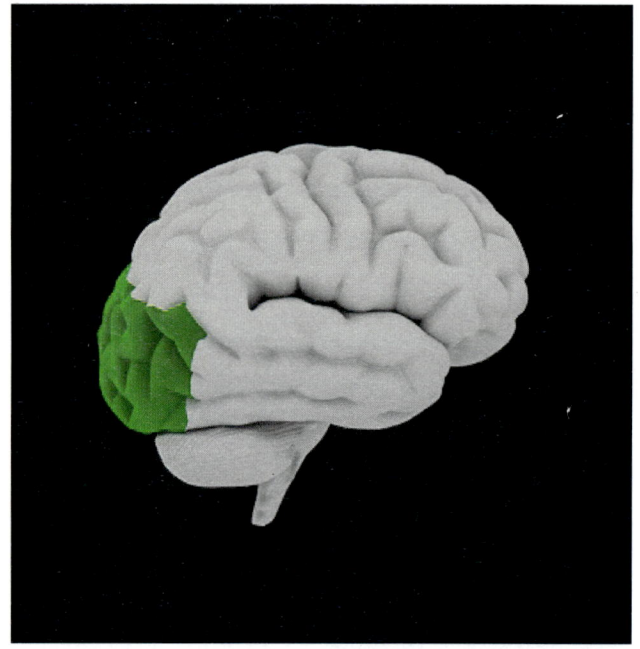

Visual recognition does not solely involve perceiving letters and words. Another significant part of visual recognition is the capability to read fluently. The "letter-box" area is also stimulated when trying to determine the words with different fonts and letter cases. For example, the "letter-box" area of the occipital lobe is stimulated as it deciphers whether a word in complete uppercase is the same as the same word in complete lowercase.

The brain networks must develop the capability to recognize that a letter that is in uppercase is the same as the same letter in lowercase or in a different font. The necessity to decipher between two fonts or two different letter cases is a significant reason why one's brain networks regarding the occipital lobe must be matured in order to read effectively and fluently.

The Effect on Dyslexics

Those with dyslexia, however, can have challenges with either the ability to perceive speech sounds quickly and accurately or the ability to perceive written letters quickly and accurately. If a dyslexic has challenges with identification and perceiving written letters, or visual recognition then, the "letter-box" area does not respond in the same way it does for typical readers to written word stimuli. Good readers show a well-developed "letterbox" area; however, dyslexics show no such maturation of the "letter-box" area for written words.

The dyslexic brain shows a disorganized circuitry. In the majority of dyslexics, the phonological or sound circuitry of the left hemisphere is subtly chaotic, and disorganization causes failure to learn proper interconnection of visual letter recognition with speech sounds. The dyslexics "letter-box" area does not develop fully nor at the "normal" speed. Dyslexics' responses to single-word identification in the left cortex of their brain are less compared to that of good readers. Dyslexics with visual recognition challenges have difficulty reading fluently and effectively because their brain, specifically their "letter-box" area, is not as mature to that of a good reader. For a dyslexic reader, there are not enough brain networks to send signals to properly identify word stimuli. Therefore, brain networks and gray and white matter in the brain must be built to develop and mature the brain so the dyslexic can effectively and fluently read.

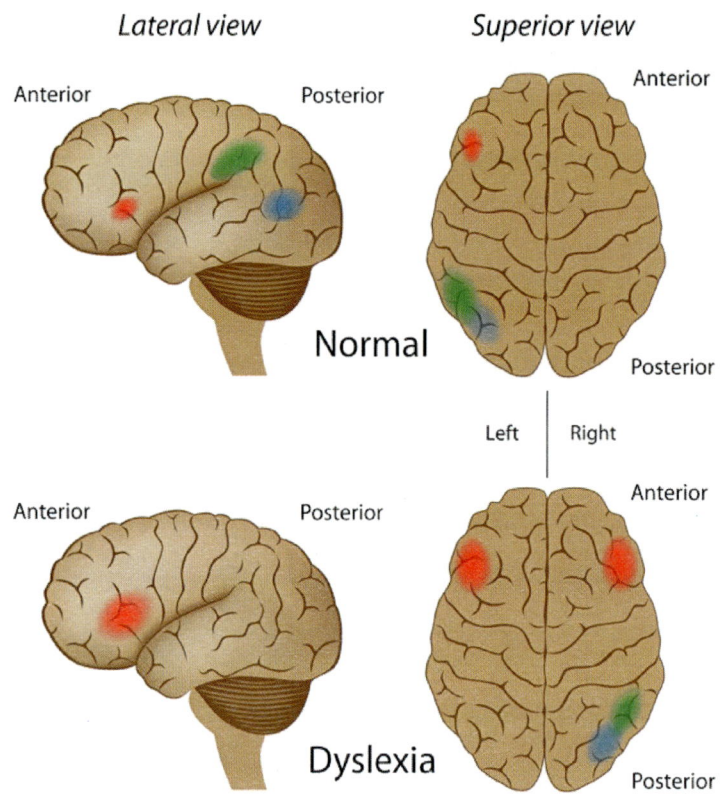

Curative Actions

In order to best remedy the lack of visual word formation abilities, reading interventions using letters, small words, and eventually large words are found to increase both white matter and gray matter quantities in the brain, therefore developing more brain networks in order to send signals quicker and fluently and effectively read. The following exercises can help develop the skills needed to increase the amount of brain networks to mature the brain for fluent reading and accurate visual recognition. Each level of exercise gets increasingly more challenging to strengthen that skill.

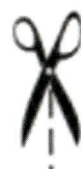

Visual Recognition: Level 1

Instructions: These exercises involve recognition of a single letter. For this exercise, please put a check next to the word that best corresponds to the image on the left of the words.

1.   (Put a ✔ next to the correct word)

	dog	
	bog	

2.

	quaint	
	paint	

3.

	nose	
	uose	

4.

	iadybug	
	ladybug	

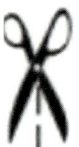

5.

	sand	
	zand	

6.

	jaguar	
	iaguar	

7.

	ball	
	pall	

8.

	foot	
	toot	

9.

	nonkey	
	monkey	

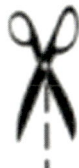

10.

	house	
	nouse	

11.

	ymbrella	
	umbrella	

12.

	goat	
	yoat	

13.

	mheel	
	wheel	

14.

	cane	
	oane	

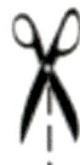

Visual Recognition: Level 2

Instructions: These exercises involve recognition of multiple letters or words. For this exercise, please put a check next to the word that best corresponds to the image on the left of the words.

1.   (Put a ✔ next to the correct word)

	<u>no</u>	
	<u>on</u>	

2.

	b**<u>ee</u>**	
	b**<u>y</u>**	

3.

	b**<u>are</u>**	
	b**<u>ear</u>**	

4.

	ang**<u>le</u>**	
	ang**<u>el</u>**	

5.

	ga**t**or	
	ta**g**or	

6.

	f<u>**in**</u>**d**	
	f<u>**rie**</u>**nd**	

7.

	fe**l**t	
	le**f**t	

8.

	pit	
	tip	

9.

	sa**w**	
	wa**s**	

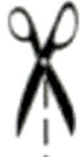

10.

	child	
	chidl	

11.

	reserve	
	reverse	

12.

	dairy	
	diary	

13.

	quite	
	quiet	

14.

	rain	
	reign	

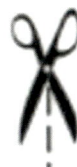

Visual Recognition: Level 3

Instructions: These exercises involve recognition of multiple letters or words. For this exercise, please put a check next to the word that best corresponds to the image on the left of the words.

1.   (Put a ✔ next to the correct word)

	pasghetti	
	spaghetti	

2.

	ci**min**on	
	ci**nnam**on	

3.

	p**ear**	
	p**air**	

4.

	left	
	right	

5.

| | h**are** | |
| | h**air** | |

6.

| | **al**o**ne** | |
| | **a** lo**an** | |

7.

| | ta**le** | |
| | ta**il** | |

8.

| | n**un** | |
| | **none** | |

9.

| | **item** | |
| | **time** | |

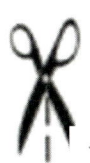

10.

	name	
	mane	

11.

	br**ake**	
	br**eak**	

12.

	wa**ste**	
	wa**ist**	

13.

	st**air**	
	st**are**	

14.

	cereal	
	serial	

Section I Lesson 2: Visual Memory

Overview

Visual memory is a type of memory which retains characteristics pertaining to our visual senses. Examples of mental images that our visual memory stores include objects, places, and faces. Visual memory has a long term and a short term. For example, some can remember people's faces over the span of many years. Short-term visual memory includes constant eye movements and the things seen during those eye movements. Short-term visual memory is usually stored for no longer than 30 seconds. For example, when driving, one's eyes are always moving. However, not all of the objects or people seen are remembered. The human brain only stores a minute amount of the information one sees and processes. Visual memory helps with comprehension and spelling, as many people visualize the word in their head as it is spelled when they are told to spell a word. Visual memory helps with comprehension because for some, when reading or listening to a passage, they visualize what is happening in their heads so they comprehend the information better. There are many things that can impact one's visual memory, like, sleep, alcohol, age, or brain damage.

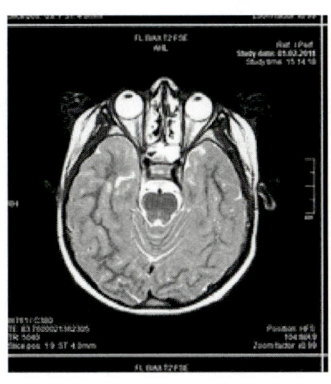 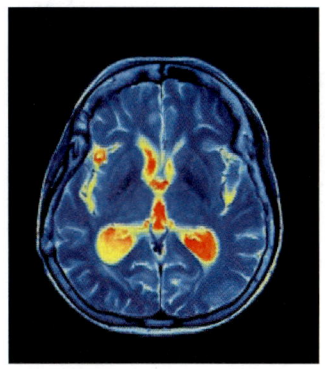

The Science: The Brain and Memory

The human brain is divided into many different areas. Areas that are specialized for visual object memory lie in the temporal cortex inferior to the ventral stream and the parietal cortex superior to the dorsal stream. The dorsal and the ventral stream maintain intercommunication during the whole course, so none of the information is lost when processing it. The dorsal stream is mainly concerned with the location of objects outside of the body. The dorsal stream is also commonly termed the "where" passage. The "where" passage begins in the occipital lobe with solely visual information, then transfers that information to the parietal cortex for that information to be stored and used for spatial awareness functions. Within the parietal cortex, there is a posterior parietal lobe which controls motor and sensory portions of the brain and manipulates mental images. The posterior parietal lobe controls the majority of the attention-based actions that the body performs. Therefore, attention and visual awareness/memory should be differentiated because, although they take place in similar locations, they do not utilize the common processes or behaviors.

However, the ventral stream pathway, commonly referred to as the "what" pathway, is mainly involved in object recognition. The ventral stream also starts at the occipital lobe with raw visual information, then transfers information to the temporal lobe for the information to be stored, processed, and analyzed by adding an emotion relating the object.

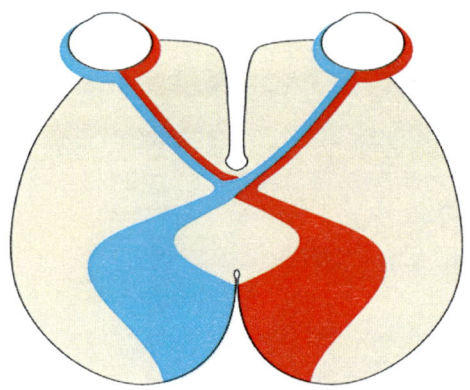 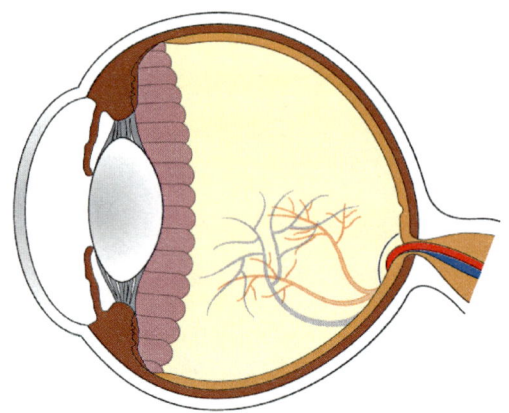

The Effect on Dyslexics

Dyslexics that have challenges with visual memory also tend to have challenges with spelling, recognizing words by sight, and navigating to unknown locations using visual cues. Dyslexics with this difficulty also have challenges with spelling because, in the English language, many words are irregular and do not follow common phonetic rules. The only way to know how to spell those irregular words is by using visual memory, to memorize how the word looks spelled out, therefore to reproduce the same spelling.

Dyslexics also have difficulty recognizing words by sight because usually, they do not memorize what the words are based on sight, instead using phonics. Therefore, dyslexics commonly have challenges with reading fluently because they forget how the word is spelled and ultimately the identity of the word itself. The part of the dyslexic brain is not stimulated upon seeing visual cues, and the information is therefore not properly processed.

Curative Actions

The best way to effectively, efficiently, and accurately improve one's visual memory and train one's brain to stimulate and memorize new information is by practicing with repetition. Many students in middle school are taught to handwrite a sentence many times to memorize it, and subconsciously the student is retaining that information into his/her longterm visual memory. In order to increase visual memory with shapes, objects, faces, and places, the thing being memorized should also be shown with variations in orientation and concentration. The following exercises can help develop the skills needed in order to increase the amount of brain networks to mature the brain for the maximum amount of visual memory abilities. Each level of exercise gets increasingly more challenging to strengthen that skill.

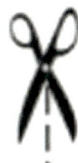

Visual Memory: Level 1

Instructions: For this exercise, please have a timer. Set the timer for 20 seconds and try to memorize every item in the image below. You are not allowed to take notes during the 20 seconds. Once the 20 seconds are completed, turn the page and write down all the items you remember seeing. Once the 20 seconds are done, you cannot go back and look at the image again.

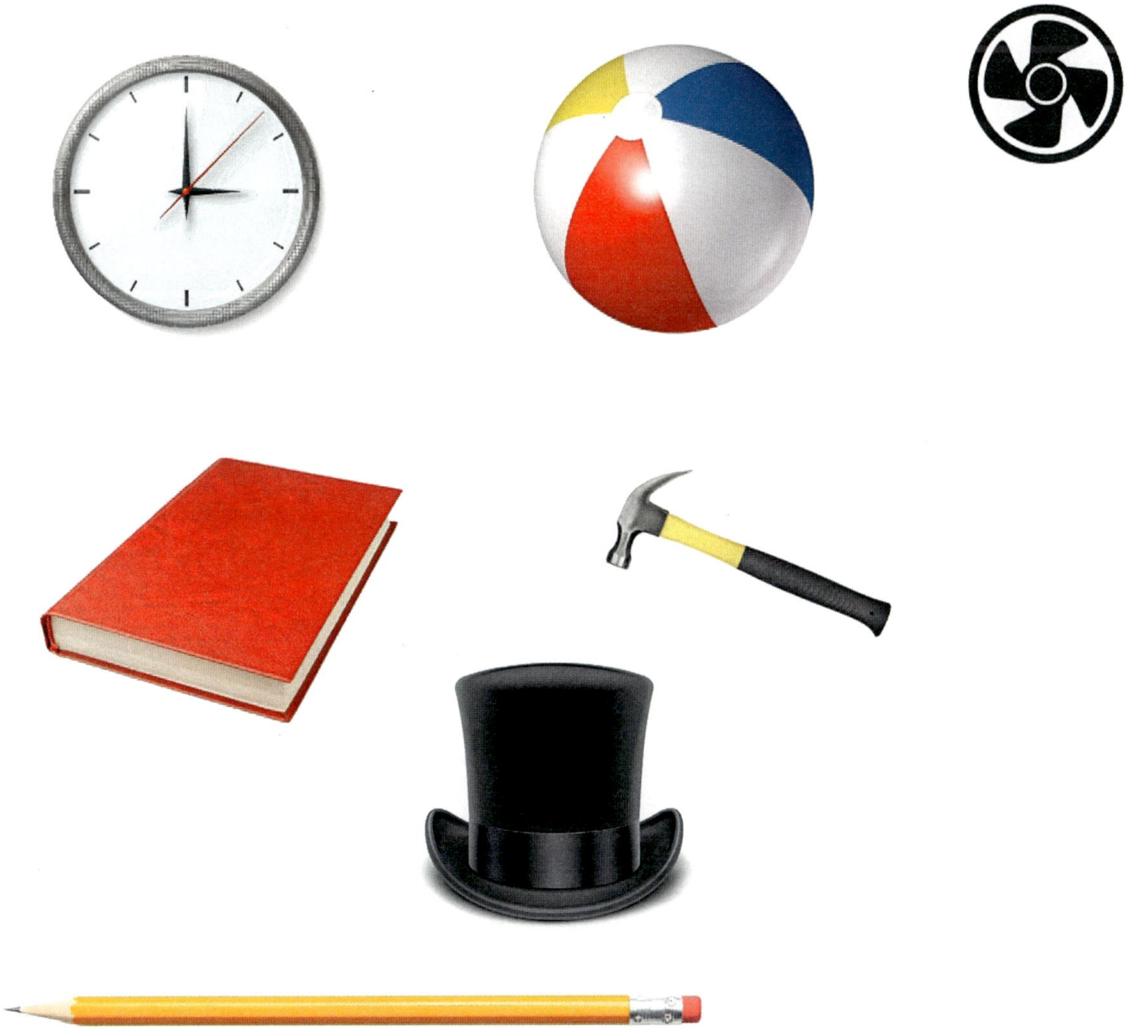

1. _____

2. _____

3. _____

4. _____

5. _____

6. _____

7. _____

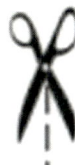

Visual Memory: Level 2

Instructions: For this exercise, please have a timer. Set the timer for 30 seconds and try to memorize every item in the image below. You are not allowed to take notes during the 30 seconds. Once the 30 seconds are completed, turn the page and write down all the items you remember seeing. Once the 30 seconds are done, you cannot go back and look at the image again.

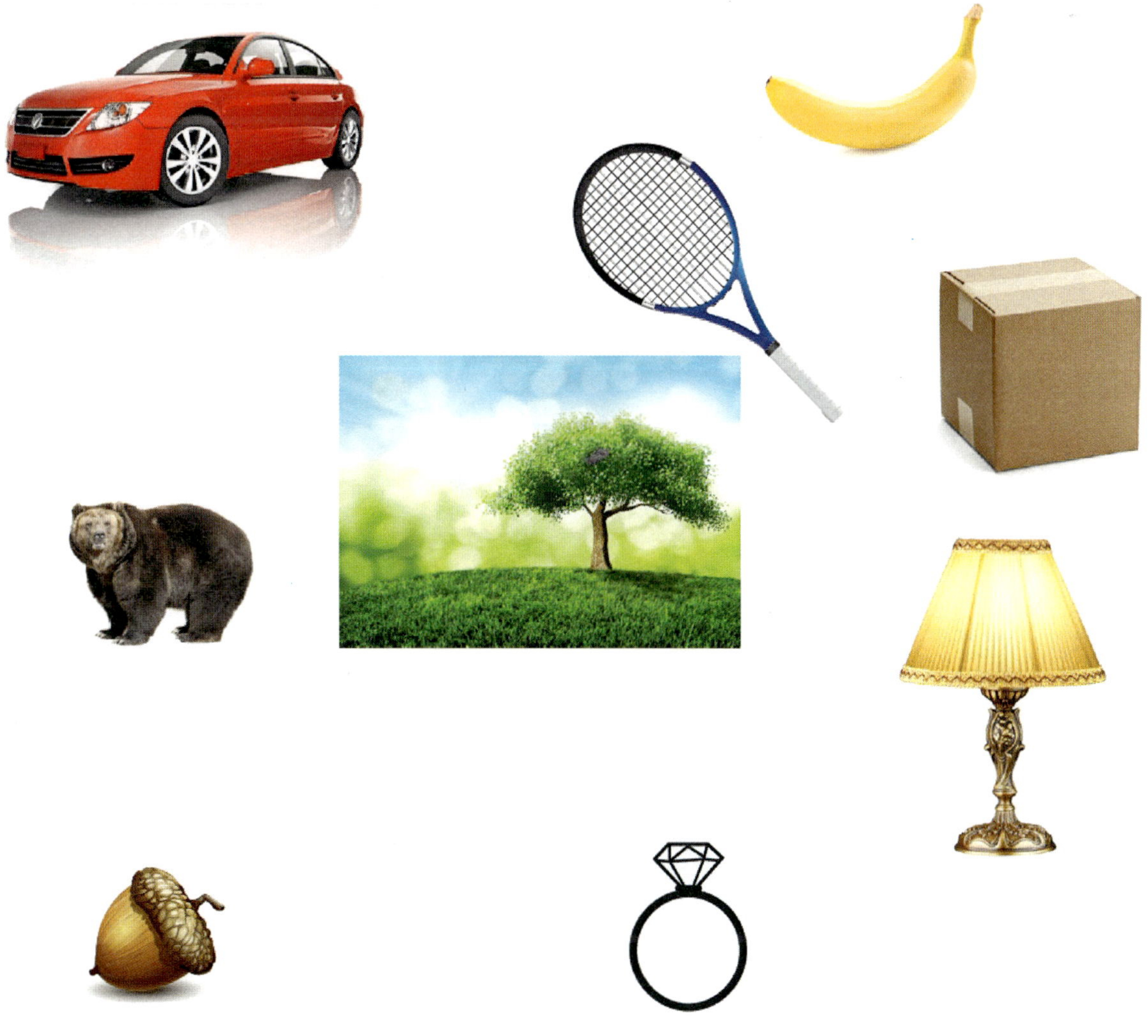

1. _____

2. _____

3. _____

4. _____

5. _____

6. _____

7. _____

8. _____

9. _____

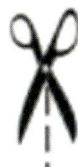

Visual Memory: Level 3

Instructions: For this exercise, please have a timer. Set the timer for 40 seconds and try to memorize every item in the image below. You are not allowed to take notes during the 40 seconds. Once the 40 seconds are completed, turn the page and write down all the items you remember seeing. Once the 40 seconds are done, you cannot go back and look at the image again.

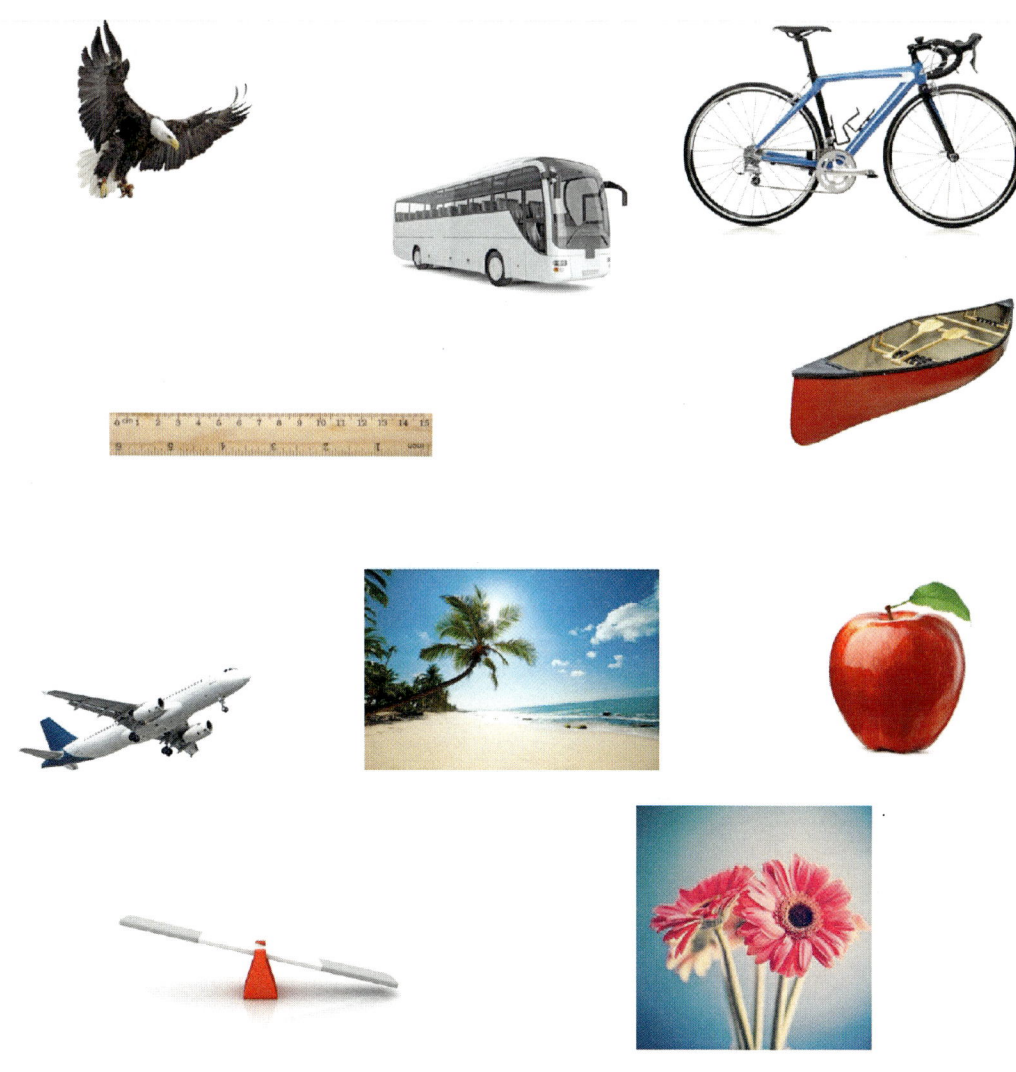

1. _____

2. _____

3. _____

4. _____

5. _____

6. _____

7. _____

8. _____

9. _____

10. _____

Section I Lesson 3: Visual Sequencing

Overview

Visual sequencing is the ability to see or picture objects in a particular order. Visual sequencing is a major factor in visual processing, the retention and comprehension of words. Visual sequencing also helps with fluent writing as the order of words in a sentence depend heavily on sequencing as well as the order of sentences in a paragraph, and even paragraphs in a writing piece. Usually, many schools teach children how to order sentences in a paragraph, but subconsciously, the teachers are helping to develop the children's brain and sequential abilities, and also training the children to learn how to effectively sequence things on their own. Visual sequencing is often taught. However, it can be naturally developed at an older age, if not initially taught to a child at a young age. Visual sequencing also has relation to one's ability to clearly follow a set of given directions. A dyslexic who has difficulty with visual sequencing will mix up, add, or omit one or more directions, because they are lacking the skills of building and storing areas to retain, perceive, and act upon the information they are given.

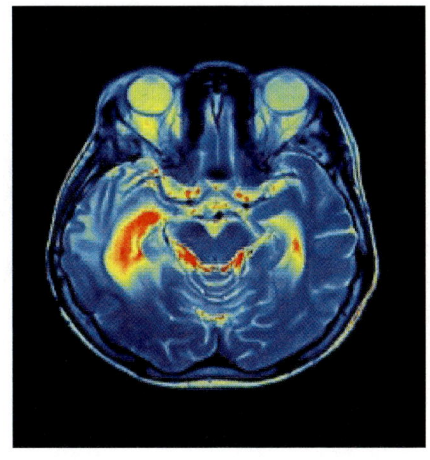

The Science: The Brain and Sequencing

The area of the brain that is affected for visual sequencing is the parietal, temporal, and occipital lobe. The back base part of one's brain, the occipital lobe is responsible for getting raw visual information. Once processed, the information is transferred to the parietal lobe, which is largely used for language and construction ability. In addition to visual sequencing, the parietal lobe also controls visual perception and spatial perception. The temporal lobes, located on the sides of the human brain, is the final location where sequential information is stored. In the temporal lobes, the information is put in the long-term, short-term, or working memory, and the information to perform actions are sent to the body. The temporal lobe also controls the body's sense of organization and is where the information for sequencing takes the most amount of time. The brain remembers all of the relevant sequencing, like how to walk or stand up by using "place cells". Place cells are active nerve cells that stimulate when the body moves into a certain part of the recognizable spatial environment. The brain contains millions of these place cells which can overlap and be used at the same time or in consecutive order. Each cell has its own mechanism for when it should be stimulated which is based on the raw information that is coming in from the occipital lobe in the brain.

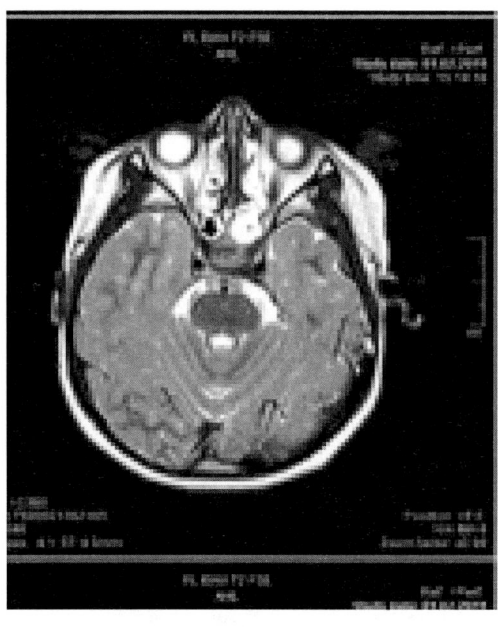

The Effect on Dyslexics

Those with dyslexia could have difficulty with their ability to visually sequence. There could be many reasons for why a dyslexic could have difficulties with visual sequencing. First, a dyslexic could have difficulty producing or storing place cells. If a dyslexic has difficulty with the ability to produce place cells, they have to repeatedly do the action in the precise sequential order in order to develop the long-term memory for how to complete that sequence. More commonly, another reason that a dyslexic has challenges with visual sequencing is that their temporal cortex is not fully developed and not all the information that the occipital lobe has is being transferred to the parietal nor the temporal lobes. Many dyslexics have challenges with both perceiving something in a sequence and remembering the sequence. These challenges are largely one of the reasons why dyslexics with visual sequencing challenges have difficulty spelling and reading because all words are letters in a specific sequence.

Curative Actions

In order to best remedy the lack of visual sequencing abilities, training and repetition will help develop more brain networks to be quicker and store more place cells to sequence information faster. The following exercises can help develop the skills needed to increase the amount of brain networks to mature the brain for fluent reading and accurate visual sequencing. Each level of exercise gets increasingly more challenging to strengthen that skill.

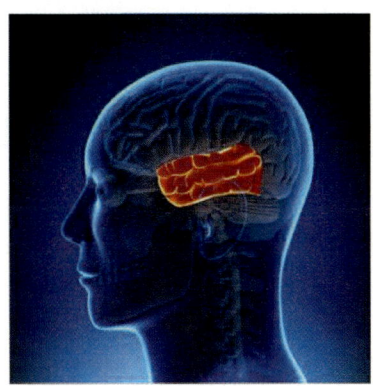

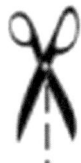

Visual Sequencing: Level 1

Instructions: For this exercise, please number the items in order from least (1) to greatest.

1.

T F R O P L W B E

_ _ _ _ _ _ _ _ _

2.

73 54 29 83 63 55 90 42 38

— — — — — — — — —

3.

Brushing teeth	Getting in your car	Eating breakfast	Waking up

_____   _____   _____   _____

Visual Sequencing: Level 2

Instructions: For this exercise, please number the items in order from least (1) to greatest.

1.

Q S R O P V T M W

___ ___ ___ ___ ___ ___ ___ ___ ___

2.

89 87.5 83 8 108 90 82 78

___ ___ ___ ___ ___ ___ ___ ___

3.

| Put on seat belt | Drive away | Lock house door | Grab car keys |

___   ___   ___   ___

4. Reorder the following letters so they make a word.

NDALAECR   _____

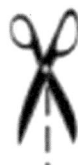

Visual Sequencing: Level 3

Instructions: For this exercise, please number the items in order from least (1) to greatest.

1.

QL QR RO OR PT PS TR

____ ____ ____ ____ ____ ____ ____

2.

51 55.5 55.55 5 505 55 0.5

____ ____ ____ __ ____ ____ ____

3.

Close house door	Open car door	Get in car	Turn on car

_____ _____ _____ _____

4. Reorder the following letters so they make a word.

KESPIROTCH _____

SMETCYHRI _____

Section II: The Sense of Hearing

Importance

Hearing is a very important human sense. Hearing is the ability to interpret sounds and receive speech which is used in order to allow humans to communicate. The hearing system detects the sound's location, pitch, and volume, among other auditory signals. Unlike what the visual system does for colors, the auditory system does not blend nor mix sounds, but separates the sounds into their base tones or components. The sound travels in waves through the ear so the pressure builds up and creates vibrations off of the eardrum. Then, the vibrations bounce off of a membrane based on the highness or lowness of its pitch. Sounds travel through the external, middle, and inner ear before it can be processed and perceived by the brain.

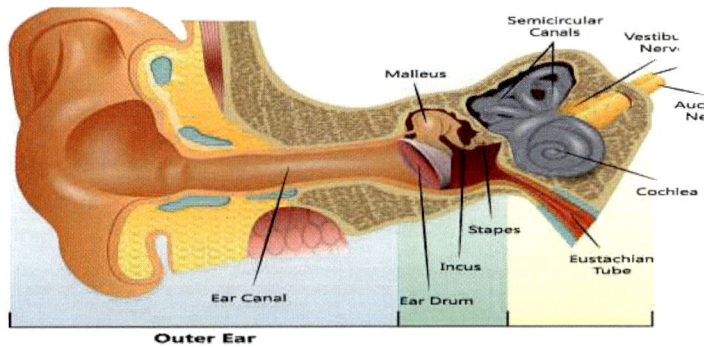

External Ear

The pinna, or outer ear, has ridges that efficiently siphons sound into the ear canal and eardrum. The pinna also helps to localize the origin of the sound. Sound waves vibrate the eardrum and cause sound energy to be sent to the middle ear.

Middle Ear

The small, air-filled middle ear is attached to the eardrum on one side and an oval window of the inner ear on the other. This air pocket is bounded by the Eustachian tube to the mouth and nasal cavity to equalize air pressure between the outside and inside of the ear. The middle ear also has the body's three smallest bones, therefore creating a pathway for vibrations to be sent from the eardrum to the inner ear.

Inner Ear

The cochlea in the inner ear has fluid that moves based on the oval window movements caused by the vibrations of the middle ear. These fluid vibrations by the cochlea cause small hair cells on the cochlea to activate, creating energy to be sent to the brain for the sound to be processed.

Auditory Exercises

The following three lessons and worksheets focus on recognition, memory, and sequencing respectively and how they impact one's reading skills and function with regards to brain activity. After each lesson there is a series of three exercise that increase in difficulty strengthen a dyslexic brain in that specific area.

Section II Lesson 4: Auditory Recognition

Overview

Auditory recognition is one's ability to perceive sounds quickly and accurately. Auditory recognition is a major component of fluent and efficient reading, as reading requires phoneme-grapheme correspondence. Phoneme- grapheme correspondence is one of the many underlying capacities needed for reading and involves the integration of sounds (phonemes) and letters (graphemes). Normally, young children develop the ability to auditorily recognize letters and words, through listening to a book read aloud. Therefore, the child's brain networks mature, so they are able to read fluently as they get older. Auditory recognition is useful when for reading, comprehending, and recognizing words that are heard.

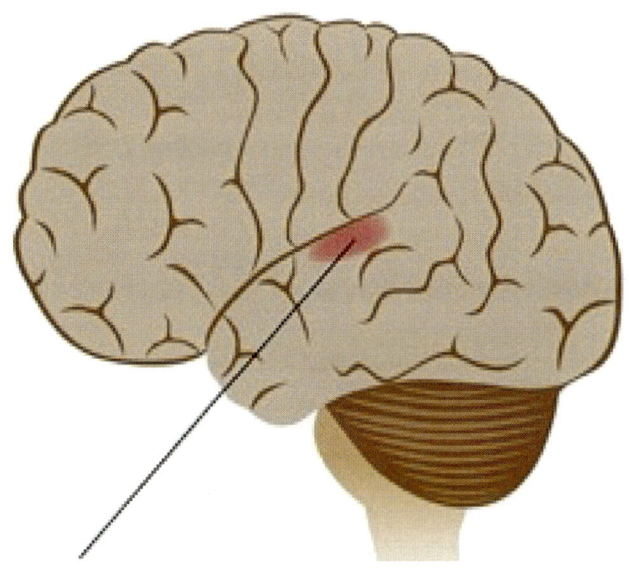

The Science: The Brain and Reading

The human brain is divided into many different areas. When the sound is heard through the ear, either one of the two layers of the cerebral cortex receives the information. At each end of the two hemispheres of the cerebral cortex, each auditory thalamus processes the previously received information. The auditory sensations are then transferred to the auditory cortex which is broken down into three separate areas: the primary, secondary, and tertiary area. These areas are concentric with the tertiary area being the outermost layer and are located in the temporal lobe approximately where the cochlea is located. The primary auditory cortex is composed of two areas named the Brodmann areas 41 and 42. It is located right above the ears. The function of the primary auditory cortex is to process sound such information as pitch, volume, and the location of a sound and is a major factor for understanding language. The secondary auditory cortex has an important role in the analysis of complex sounds and sound localization, especially for language. The secondary cortex also has a role in auditory memory. The brain, near the auditory cortex, has a layer which surrounds all three layers of the auditory cortex called the "belt region". The belt region helps to integrate hearing with the other sensory systems: touch, smell, taste, and sight.

In the auditory cortex, the sounds are finally perceived and then transfer back out to the parietal and frontal lobes of the cerebral cortex.

Within the auditory cortex, the layers of cells that receive the processed information are used to perceive natural sounds, as well as those used for communication.

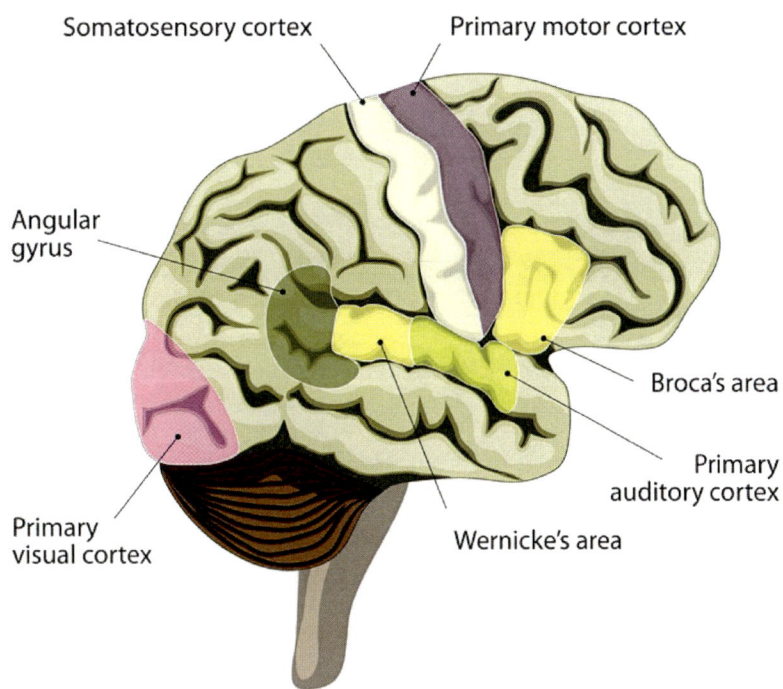

The Effect on Dyslexics

Those with dyslexia, however, can have challenges with the ability to perceive speech sounds quickly and accurately. If a dyslexic has challenges with identification and perceiving sounds or auditory recognition, then their auditory cortex area does not respond accurately to auditory stimuli. The auditory cortex area does not process the sounds of words it hears and therefore does not perceive those words to have meaning. Dyslexics often have an inability to normally process linguistic input as a result of intrahemispheric or interhemispheric connectivity abnormalities. Another area that is commonly abnormal in dyslexics with auditory recognition challenges is the parietotemporal lobe, as there are common deficits of temporal sequencing of information and interaural asymmetry in dichotic listening. Dyslexics have difficulty deriving phonological segments from the acoustic stream of speech. Components of auditory temporal processing deficit, however, claim that dyslexics with language-learning difficulties have trouble in processing sounds fast enough to distinguish rapid acoustic changes in speech.

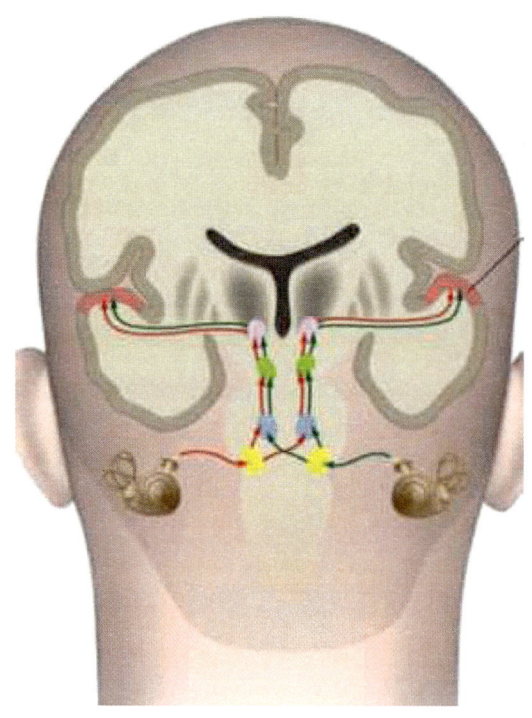

Curative Actions

In order to best remedy the lack of auditory recognizing abilities, listening interventions using letters, small words, and eventually large words are found to increase both white matter and gray matter quantities in the brain, therefore developing more brain networks and strengthen the auditory cortex in order to send signals quicker and fluently and effectively read and comprehend. The following exercises can help develop the skills needed to increase the amount of brain networks to mature the brain for fluent reading and comprehension as well as accurate auditory recognition. Each level of exercise gets increasingly more challenging to strengthen that skill.

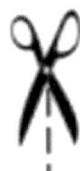

Auditory Recognition: Level 1

Instructions: These exercises involve recognition of a single letter. For this exercise, you will need help from another person. Please ask the other person to read the words below and the number that corresponds to them, then on the following two pages please circle whichever answer choice best fits the word read.

1. L
2. F
3. B
4. N
5. T
6. S
7. O
8. U
9. D
10. R

.

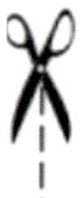

Circle the correct answer.

1.   L   J   2.   E   F

3.   B   D   4.   N   M

5.   T   I   6.   Z   S

7.   O   C   8.   U   P

9.   G   D   10.   R   P

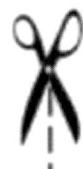

Auditory Recognition: Level 2

<u>Instructions:</u> These exercises involve recognition of a multiple letters. For this exercise, you will need help from another person. Please ask the other person to read the words or letters below and the number that corresponds to them, then on the following two pages please circle whichever answer choice best fits the word read.

1. TO

2. NAT

3. PUT

4. PIG

5. VAN

6. JET

7. SUN

8. RAM

9. SNAIL

10. MATCH

Circle the correct answer.

1.

TO   DO

2.

NAT   FAT

3.

NUT   PUT

4.

PIG   WIG

5.

FAN   VAN

6.

JET   PET

7.

SUN   RUN

8.

HAM   RAM

9.

SNAIL   TAIL

10.

PATCH   MATCH

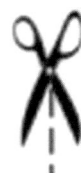

Auditory Recognition: Level 3

Instructions: These exercises involve recognition of words. For this exercise, you will need help from another person. Please ask the other person to read the words or letters below and the number that corresponds to them, then on the following two pages please circle whichever answer choice best fits the word read.

1. BALL

2. MALL

3. HIKE

4. SOAP

5. JUICE

6. BOOT

7. DRILL

8. TREE

9. PEAR

10. SHEEP

Circle the correct answer.

1.

   BALL   TALL

2.

   DOLL   MALL

3.

   BIKE   HIKE

4.

   SOAP   ROPE

5.

   JUICE   GOOSE

6.

   SUIT   BOOT

7.

   DRILL   GRILL

8.

   TREE   THREE

9.
   CHAIR   PEAR

10.
   SHEEP   SLEEP

Section II Lesson 5: Auditory Memory

Overview

Auditory memory is the ability to take in orally transmitted information, process it, retain it in one's mind, and recall it for future use. Auditory memory is important for reading comprehension and following directions carefully. When one is tasked to comprehend an oral story, they are asked to use their auditory memory to receive and process the information that they are hearing. Auditory memory requires a good working memory. Working memory is the ability to manipulate and manage information from one's short-term and long-term memory. Working memory is used for more complex and higher level linguistics. Unlike visual memory, auditory memory cannot be scanned over and over again, so there is only one chance to retain all of the possible information. Auditory memory is stored for a longer period of time than visual memory. Auditory memory uses what is known as the "holding tank" concept, which means the information received does not get processed until the following sound is received because the following sounds give the initial sound meaning. Once the initial auditory stimuli are presented, the brain replays the sound for a brief time before either processing the information or negating it. The brief time that the sound is held lasts for a mere 3-4 seconds.

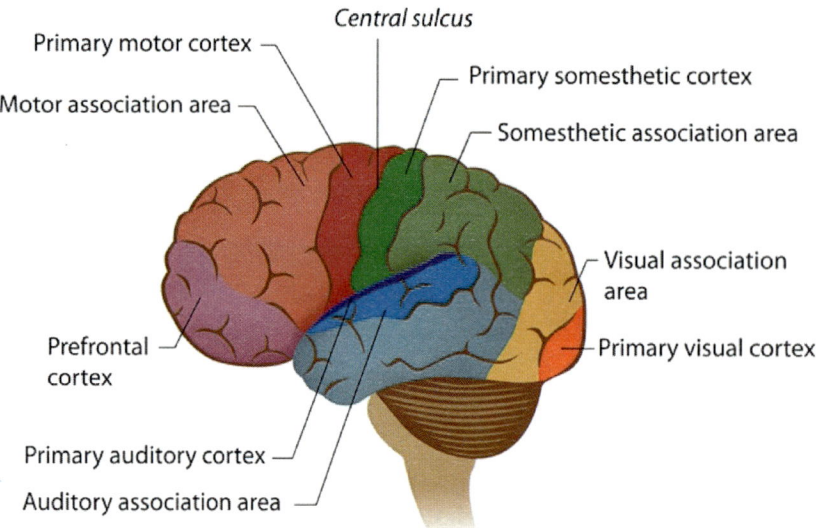

The Science: The Brain and Memory

Auditory memory is found to be in several areas of the brain because of the large amounts of processes it is involved in. However, auditory memory is stored mainly in the primary auditory cortex. Most of the areas that auditory memory processes take place in are part of the prefrontal cortex, where most of the executive control of the brain is located. The memory, rehearsal, and phonological systems are stored in the left hemisphere of the brain. However, the three major areas that are involved in auditory memory are the left posterior ventrolateral prefrontal cortex (VLPFC), the left posterior parietal cortex (PPC), and the left premotor cortex (PMC). The main location responsible for verbal rehearsal and articulatory processes is within the VLPFC and is called the Broca's area. The main location responsible for rhythmic organization and rehearsal is in the dorsal PMC, and the PPC is responsible for localizing objects based off of sound proximity in space. In addition, some stimulation has been seen in the superior temporal gyrus (STG) and the inferior temporal gyrus (ITG) when processes of auditory memory have been activated.

The Effect on Dyslexics

Dyslexics that have challenges with auditory memory, most likely have an atypical structure of their primary auditory cortex. The neuroanatomical region of the auditory cortex, in general, has a strong cortical thickness protecting this sensory area. Those with dyslexia may differ significantly in the thickness of the cortical protective area. Executive control and sensory processes could differ in a child that does not have adequate amounts of cortical protection around their sensory cortex. In this instance, cortical inadequacies could result in challenges regarding auditory memory, and could, therefore, be the result of difficulties with reading, comprehension, and other auditory sensory challenges. These sensory difficulties could also discourage the dyslexic from reading, as weak cortical protective areas could make learning to read more effortful, despite proper teaching, and when the dyslexic reads, they might lack the comprehension of the passage after rereading it multiple times. Those with dyslexia show impaired and slower amplitude modulations compared to those without dyslexia. Adult dyslexics also show neuronal impairment to higher volumes and pitches with differences sourced from the primary auditory cortex. This demonstrates that those with dyslexia lack auditory memory if what they are told is within a certain range of volume and pitch. As the age of the dyslexic increases, so does the range of volume and pitch that the dyslexic can process.

Curative Actions

In order to best remedy the lack of auditory memory abilities, listening interventions using letters, small words, and eventually large words are found to increase both the thickness of the protection surrounding the auditory cortex there strengthening the signals that are transferred to the auditory cortex to be stored. The following exercises can help develop the skills needed to increase the amount of brain networks to mature the brain for fluent reading and comprehension as well as accurate auditory recognition. Each level of exercise gets increasingly more challenging to strengthen that skill.

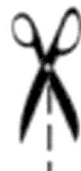

Auditory Memory: Level 1

Instructions: For this exercise, you will need help from another person. Please ask the other person to read the letters below aloud next to you. Once finished reading the letters, please wait with the book closed for 10 seconds. Once the 10 seconds are finished, then return to the book to the following page and rewrite as many of the letters in the correct order as you remember. After reading question one, wait the 10 seconds and answer it, then continue to do the same for questions two and three.

1. A F B N M Q

2. H Y W P C D S X

3. K T E G I J L O R

Please rewrite the letters here.

1. 6 Letters: _____ _____ _____ _____ _____

_____

2. 8 Letters: _____ _____ _____ _____ _____ _____

_____ _____

3. 9 Letters: _____ _____ _____ _____ _____ _____

_____ _____ _____

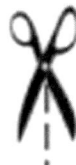

Auditory Memory: Level 2

Instructions: For this exercise, you will need help from another person. Please ask the other person to read the words below aloud next to you. Once finished reading the letters, please wait with the book closed for 10 seconds. Once the 10 seconds are finished, then return to the book to the following page and rewrite as many of the letters in the correct order as you remember. After reading question one, wait the 10 seconds and answer it, then continue to do the same for questions two and three.

1. Blue Apple Nine Note Phone Fan
2. Shield Box Elevator Sun Map Pencil Tape Water
3. Lock Orange Wolf Book Helmet Football Card Notebook Folder

Please rewrite the letters here.

1. 6 Letters: _____ _____ _____ _____ _____
_____

2. 8 Letters: _____ _____ _____ _____ _____ _____
_____ _____

3. 9 Letters: _____ _____ _____ _____ _____ _____
_____ _____ _____

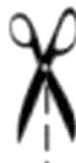

Auditory Memory: Level 3

Instructions: For this exercise, you will need help from another person. Please ask the other person to read the passage below aloud next to you, then on the following page please write as much of the passage as you remember as close to the context and similar vocabulary.

Thomas woke up one morning and look out his window. He noticed that there was a deer in his front yard. Thomas did not know what to do, so he went about the rest of his morning normally. Thomas brushed his teeth and got ready for work. Once Thomas finished his getting ready for work, he took his coffee and went to his car to drive for work. Before leaving his driveway, Thomas realized that the deer had left, but he continued to drive to work. Once Thomas arrived at work, he received a call from his wife from their house. His wife said that there were five deer eating and sleeping in their backyard. Thomas was relieved to know that the deer he saw in the morning was safe, but worried about what to do with the five deer in his backyard!

Section II Lesson 6: Auditory Sequencing

Overview

Auditory sequencing is the ability to hear and organize objects in a particular order. Auditory sequencing is a major factor in auditory processing, retention, and comprehension of sounds. Auditory sequencing also helps with comprehension and following directions as the order of directions and order of a story depend heavily on sequencing. In addition, auditory sequencing has a direct correlation to auditory memory and are located in very similar areas. Usually, many schools teach children how to follow a given sequential order, but subconsciously, the teachers are helping to develop the child's brain and sequential abilities, and also training the student to learn how to effectively sequence things on their own. Auditory sequencing is often taught. However, it can also be naturally developed at an older age, if not initially taught to the child at a younger age. Auditory sequencing also has relation to one's ability to clearly follow a set of given directions. A dyslexic who has difficulty with auditory sequencing will mix up, add, or omit one or more directions, because they lack the storing areas to retain, perceive, and act upon the information they are given.

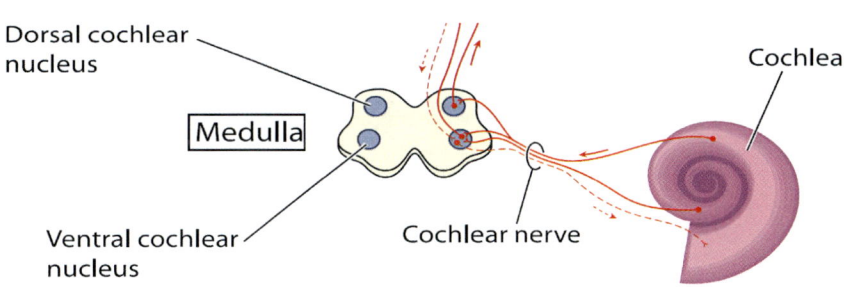

The Science: The Brain and Sequencing

The human brain is divided into many different areas. The area of the brain that is affected for auditory sequencing is the parietal, temporal, and auditory cortex lobe. The auditory sensations are then transferred to the auditory cortex which is broken down into three separate areas: the primary, secondary, and tertiary area. These areas are concentric with the tertiary area being the outermost layer and are located in the temporal lobe approximately where the cochlea is located. The primary auditory cortex is composed of two areas named the Brodmann areas 41 and 42. It is located right above the ears. In the auditory cortex, the sounds are perceived and then transfer back out to the temporal and frontal lobes of the cerebral cortex. Within the auditory cortex, the layers of cells that receive the processed information are used to perceive natural sounds, as well as those used for communication.

The temporal lobe, located on the sides of the human brain, is the final location where sequential information is stored. In the temporal lobe, the information is put in the long-term, short-term, or working memory, and the actions to perform the sequence are sent to the body. The temporal lobe also controls the body's sense of organization and is where the information for sequencing takes the most amount of time. The brain remembers all of the relevant sequencings like how to walk or stand up by using "place cells". Place cells are nerve cells that stimulate when the body moves into a certain part of the recognizable spatial environment. The brain contains millions of these place cells, and the place cells can overlap

and be used at the same time or in consecutive order. Each cell has its own mechanism for when it should be stimulated, and that is based on the raw information that is coming in from the auditory cortex of the brain.

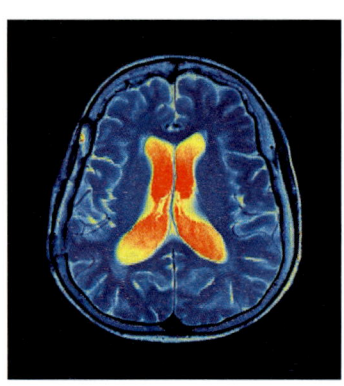

The Effect on Dyslexics

Those with dyslexia could have difficulty with their ability to auditorily sequence. There could be many reasons for why a dyslexic would have difficulties with auditory sequencing. First, a dyslexic could have difficulty producing or storing place cells. If a dyslexic has difficulty with the ability to produce place cells, he/she would have to repeatedly do the action in the precise sequential order in order to develop the long-term memory for how to complete that sequence. More commonly, another reason that a dyslexic has challenges with auditory sequencing is that their temporal cortex is not fully developed, and not all the information that the auditory cortex has is being transferred to the parietal nor the temporal lobes. Many dyslexics have challenges with both perceiving something in a sequence and remembering the sequence. These challenges are largely one of the reasons why dyslexics with visual sequencing challenges have difficulty spelling and reading because all words are letters in a specific sequence.

Curative Actions

In order to best remedy the lack of auditory sequencing abilities, training and repetition will help develop brain networks to be quicker and store more place cells to sequence information faster. The following exercises can help develop the skills needed to increase the amount of brain networks and mature the brain for precise reading comprehension and accurate auditory sequencing. Each level of exercise gets increasingly more challenging to strengthen that skill.

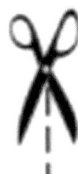

Auditory Sequencing: Level 1

Instructions: For this exercise, you will need help from another person. Please ask the other person to read the letters below aloud next to you, then on the following page please rewrite the letters so that the letters make a coherent word. Please also add the appropriate grammar markings.

1. **RIPSGN**
2. **SASRG**
3. **LOPILW**
4. **AETTS**
5. **OHSOCL**

1. _____

2. _____

3. _____

4. _____

5. _____

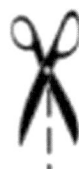

Auditory Sequencing: Level 2

Instructions: For this exercise, you will need help from another person. Please ask the other person to read the letters below aloud next to you, then on the following page please rewrite the letters so that the letters make a coherent word. Please also add the appropriate grammar markings.

VIIEESNOLT

CLLCAAURT O

GLUBDIIN

UTCERPI

NECEICS

1. _____

2. _____

3. _____

4. _____

5. _____

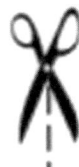

Auditory Sequencing: Level 3

Instructions: For this exercise, you will need help from another person. Please ask the other person to read the words below aloud next to you, then on the following page please rewrite the words so that the words make a coherent sentence. Please also add the appropriate grammar markings.

1. dog/ his/ owner/ the/ well/ treats

2. friend's/ I/ at/ stopped/ house/ my

3. surprise/ the/ tomorrow/ is/ party

4. broke/ charger/ my/ for/ the/ computer

5. animals/ we/ going/ see/ are/ to

1. _____

2. _____

3. _____

4. _____

5. _____

Section III: Spatial Perception

Importance

Spatial perception is the ability to understand the relationship of one's body orientation and space. It involves many characteristics, like the ability to perceive motion, position, spatial features, and spatial properties. Spatial perception is very important regarding reading, as well as normal actions. Spatial perception is also correlated with the skills such as visual-spatial relationships, visual sequencing, and visual memory. Often times, when dyslexics have difficulty with visual sequencing, memory, or recognition, they also have challenges with spatial perception as the skills needed for visual sequencing, memory, and recognition are also commonly needed for spatial perception abilities. In addition, spatial perception also involves giving meaning to objects in space, therefore attributing perceived data to one's semantic and sensory processes. Accurate spatial perception is characterized by fast and accurate performance in identification and peripheral tasks while also completing a central search, similar to intense multitasking.

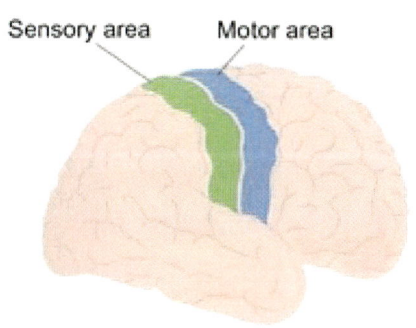

Human Position

Human position refers to one's body in space and its relation to other objects in space. Human striated skeletal muscles are equipped with proprioceptors which helps one perceive and sense body position and movement by sending off two types of signals: exteroception and interoception. Exteroception is what one senses about the outside world, while interoception is what one senses about what is happening inside one's body, like hunger or pain. This data is integrated to a vestibular system.

Reading

Spatial perception involves reading because reading uses the ability to receive and perceive the letters and words as it is written or said, thus the orientation of the letter and words and how the body understands or takes in the information results in how the sentence or word in perceived. Therefore, fluent reading and comprehension heavily depends on the ability to receive and perceive the letters and words as they are said or read.

Spatial Exercises

The following two lessons focus on body perception and spatial orientation and how they impact one's reading skills and function with regards to brain activity. After each lesson there is a series of three exercises that increase in difficulty strengthen a dyslexic brain in that specific area.

Section III Lesson 7: Body Perception

Overview

Body perception is a broad topic and is usually impacted for dyslexics. There are three kinds of body perceptions. First, internal perception, or proprioception, is based on what is occurring in our bodies. For example, proprioception tells us where are limbs are and whether we are standing, sitting, or lying down. Secondly, sensory perception, or exteroception, is based on the space and world outside our bodies. Sensory perception depends heavily on our senses of vision, touch, taste, smell, and hearing, and allows us to perceive sounds, textures, odors, and colors. This is also referred to as cognitive psychology. Lastly, mixed internal and external perception is based upon what is occurring inside our bodies and about the cause of those feelings by outside forces. This kind of perception is used for emotions and certain kinds of moods. The perceptions that are most impacted for dyslexics are sensory perceptions and internal perceptions. These perceptions do not usually differ greatly between dyslexics and non-dyslexics. However, it usually is still impacted.

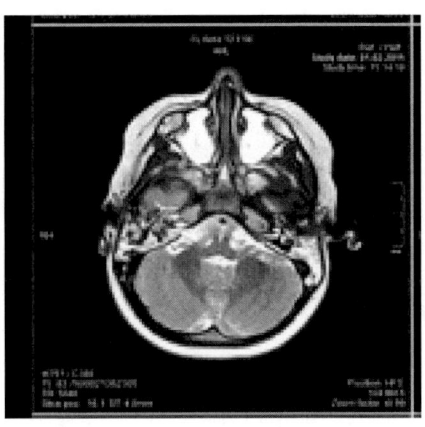

The Science: The Brain and Perceptions

There are many ways that information gets transferred into the brain for it to be processed and perceived. First, light reflects off of an object at some distance, and some rays of the light will fall upon the cornea of the eyes where two images will be formed by the retina, one by each eye. The two images will be transferred to the visual cortex, in the occipital lobe. There, two slightly different images will be processed and condensed into one image. The image will be colored and moved like the original object by parts of the visual cortex. This final image is called a "perception". Next, the image is sent to the temporal cortex via the dorsal and ventral stream. The dorsal and the ventral stream maintain intercommunication during the whole course so none of the information is lost when processing it. The dorsal stream is mainly concerned with the location of objects in the outside world. The dorsal stream is also commonly termed the "where" passage. The data is then stored in the temporal lobe until it is again needed. Another way for data to reach the brain is through the ear. Sounds are received through pressure waves in the cochlea of the ear. The auditory sensations are then transferred to the auditory cortex which is broken down into three separate areas: the primary, secondary, and tertiary area. These areas are concentric with the tertiary area being the outermost layer and are located in the temporal lobe. The primary auditory cortex is composed of two areas named the Brodmann areas 41 and 42. It is located right above the ears. The function of the primary auditory cortex is to process sounds such as pitch, volume and the location of a sound. The secondary auditory cortex has an important role in the analysis of complex sounds and sound localization, especially for language. The data that was received and processed is then transferred to the auditory cortex to be perceived. The final, perceived auditory data is then "bounded" to the final visual image in a process called the "binding problem". After the visual and auditory data is bonded, the combined data is transferred to the parietal lobe, specifically the parietal cortex. Within the parietal cortex, there is a posterior parietal lobe which controls motor and sensory portions of the brain and manipulates mental perceptions and sounds. The posterior parietal lobe controls the majority of the attention based and bodily perceptual actions that the body performs.

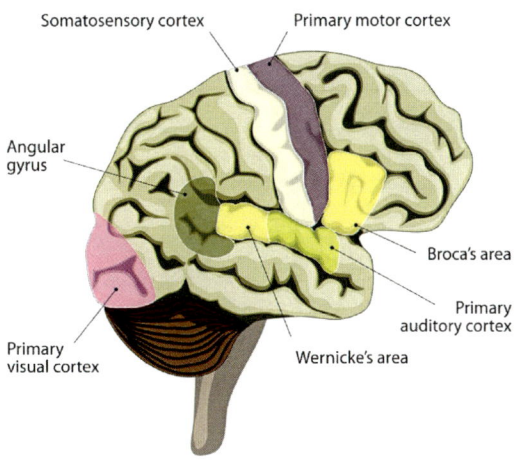

The Effect on Dyslexics

Dyslexics commonly have challenges with visuospatial bodily perception. These challenges may manifest in letter identification, the

recalling of sequences, or memorization. These perceptual difficulties that dyslexics experience could be the result of many different underlying causes. Some of these causes include visual recognition, memory, or sequencing difficulties, or auditory recognition, memory, or sequencing challenges.

Curative Actions

One of the best ways to remedy the lack of bodily perceptual abilities is by practicing with identifying body parts to develop the skills to accurately and quickly use and identify them when tasked with perceptual problems. The following exercises can help develop the skills needed to increase the speed and accuracy of brain networks to mature the brain for making precise and systematic bodily perceptions. Each level of exercise gets increasingly more challenging to strengthen that skill

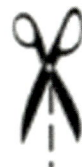

Body Perception: Level 1

Instructions: For this exercise, please match the words in the box below to the spaces on the diagram, then write the corresponding word to that space in the lines provided on the diagram. Some words may be used once, more than once, or not at all.

Left leg	Right hand	Right knee	Mouth	Chest Foot
Forehead	Left ear	Stomach	Thigh	Neck Toe

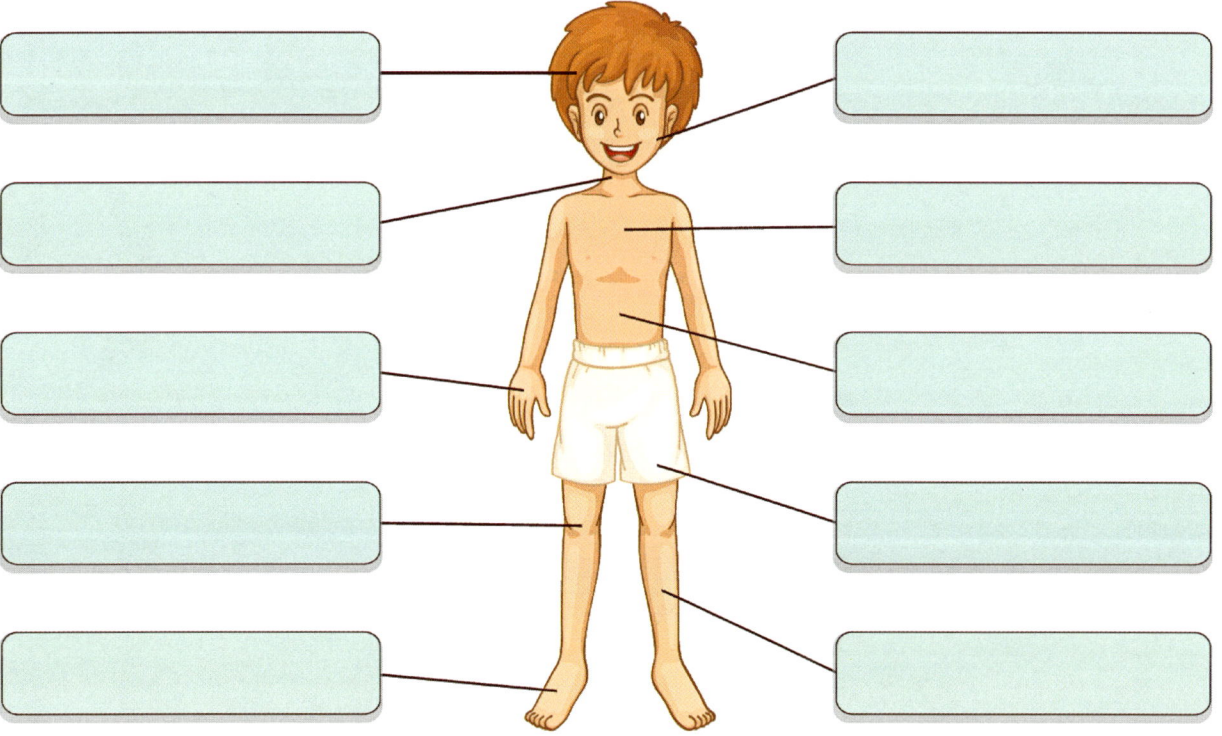

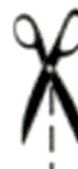

Body Perception: Level 2

Instructions: For this exercise, please match the words in the box below to the spaces on the diagram, then write the corresponding word to that space in the lines provided on the diagram. Some words may be used once, more than once, or not at all.

Computer	Monitor	Mouse pad	Printer	Copier
Mouse	Keyboard	Power cord	Speaker	Headphones

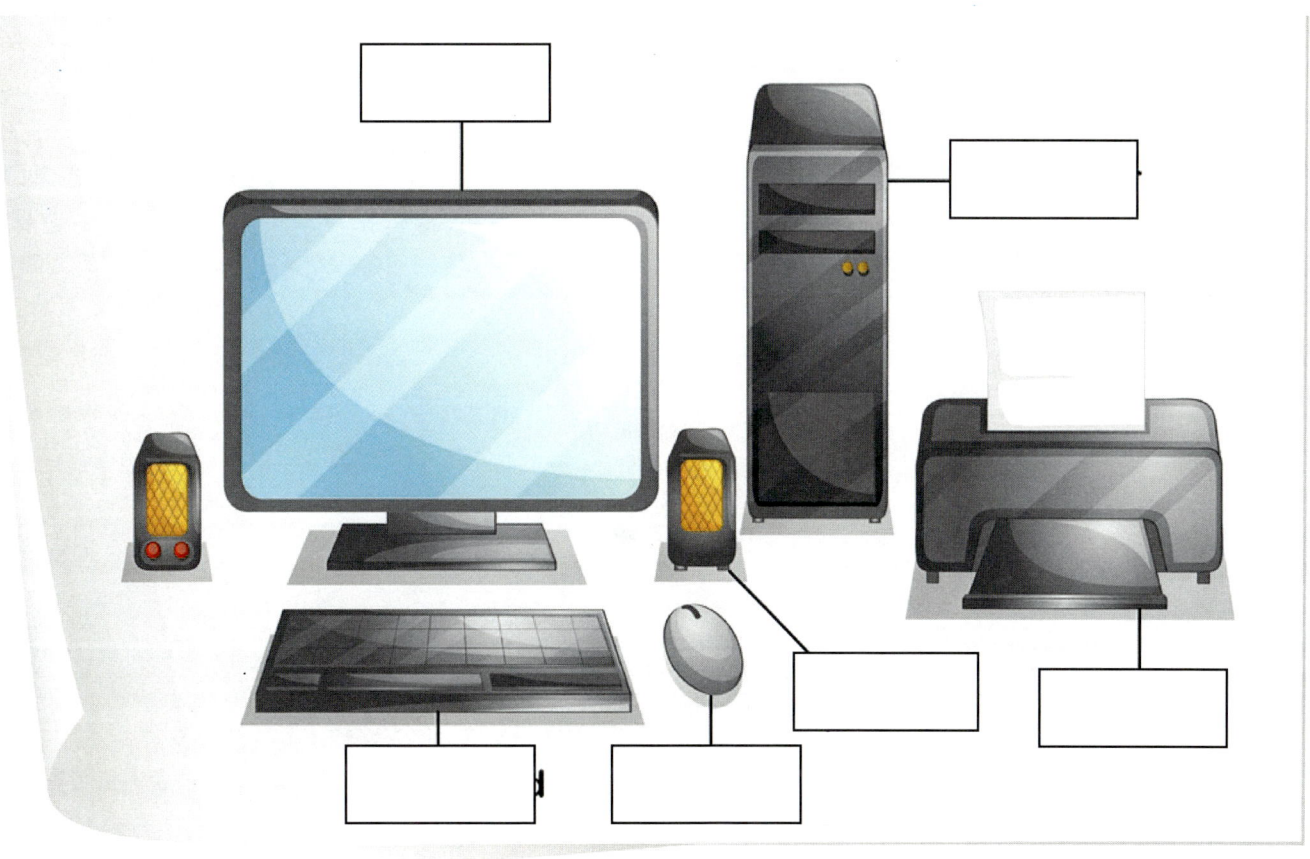

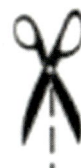

Body Perception: Level 3

Instructions: For this exercise, please match the words in the box below to the spaces on the diagram, then write the corresponding word to that space in the lines provided on the diagram. Some words may be used once, more than once, or not at all.

Headlights	Front Windshield	Seat belt	Door Steering Wheel
Hood	Windshield Wipers	Tire Rim	Tire Front Bumper

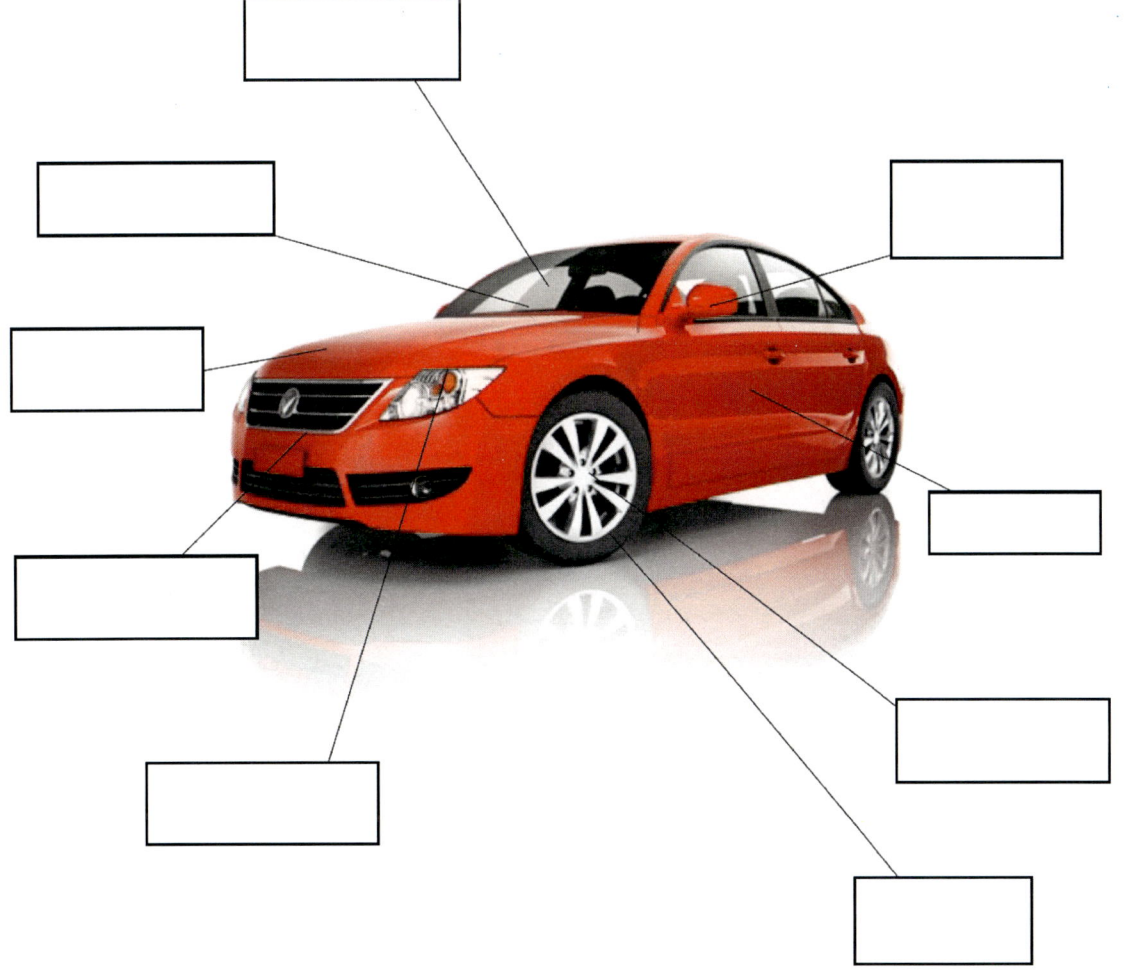

Section III Lesson 8: Spatial Orientation

Overview

Spatial orientation is one of the key abilities which must be mature early in a child's life if the child is going to learn to read and write fluently. Early in a child's life, moving patterns like crawling, rolling, rocking, and later walking and running are all important to building the child's sensory map, where the child is in space at all and any times. This is why a child is not born knowing naturally how to walk and run because the child must develop a sensory map to discover where he/she is at all times. The child develops and retains a large enough sensory map when he/she first starts to walk and run. Spatial orienting must be experienced by the child many times until it is internalized, processed, and automatic. A child learns to read and write letters in school. The child usually remembers the direction and drawing of the letters on a two-dimensional space, paper. However, some letters like D, P, B, and Q are all very similar to a child who is learning about them based off of their drawing. Therefore, it is difficult to tell them apart if the child lacks good spatial orientation skills.

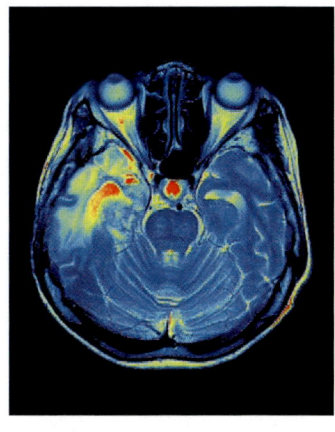

The Science: The Brain and Orientation

There are very many different areas of the brain involved with spatial orientation. First, the hippocampus in the brain provides the spatial map of one's environment. The hippocampus stores information based on reference to external cues in the environment and is context dependent. The hippocampus uses working memory to store information about spatial locations. Another location used for spatial orientation is the posterior parietal cortex. The posterior parietal cortex encodes spatial information based on data that is one's location in space. It is therefore stimulated when producing coordination actions for the body. The parietal cortex is also used for constantly updating the spatial representation of the body within its environment. Another area stimulated for spatial orientation is the dorsocaudal medial entorhinal cortex (dMEC), which contains an organized map of the spatial environment made up of grid cells. Grid cells store transformed sensory information from its environment in a durable coating. Grid cells are mainly used for path integration and navigation. In addition to the dMEC, another area in the brain used for spatial orientation includes the prefrontal cortex. The medial prefrontal cortex processes one's location in space. It is stimulated during the processing of short-term spatial memory, which is used to guide planned search behaviors. The prefrontal cortex also plays a factor in motivational significance, which is when the identification of neurons anticipates expected rewards during a spatial task. Finally, the last main area stimulated for spatial orientation is the perirhinal cortex. The perirhinal cortex is associated with both spatial reference and spatial working memory and processes relational information of environmental cues.

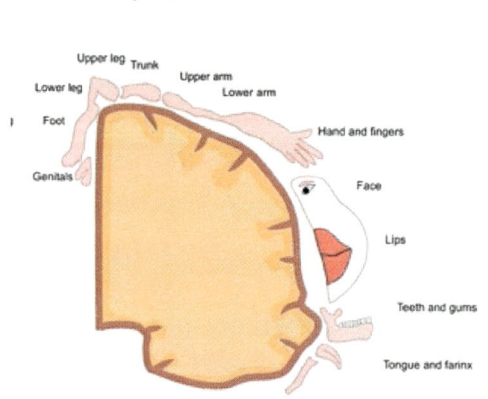

96

The Effect on Dyslexics

Children with dyslexia usually have poor spatial orientation skills. This lack of spatial orientation skills usually results in the reversal of letters after approximately age seven and poor memory of the shapes of words and other complex letters or even sounds. Asking a dyslexic child with poor spatial orientation skills to do repetitive tasks like rewriting a letter or word is pointless as the child's underlying cause lies in the brain and its development.

Curative Actions

One of the best ways to remedy the lack of spatial orientation abilities is by practicing with identifying locations and orientations to develop the skills to accurately and quickly use and identify them when tasked with orientation problems. The following exercises can help develop the skills needed to increase the speed and accuracy of brain networks to mature the brain for making precise and systematic spatial orientation. Each level of exercise gets increasingly more challenging to strengthen that skill.

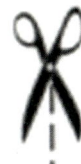

Spatial Orientation: Level 1

Instructions: For this exercise, please circle the correct answer and apply only the information given on the paper.

1. The ant is bigger than the man.

   True or False

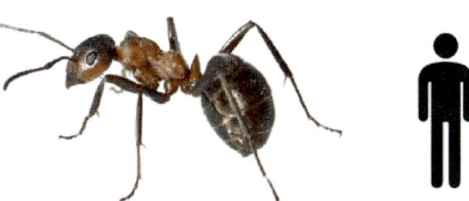

2. The letter is longer in size than the word.

   True or False

CAT

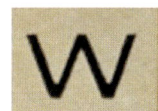

3. The panda is smaller than the snake

   True or False

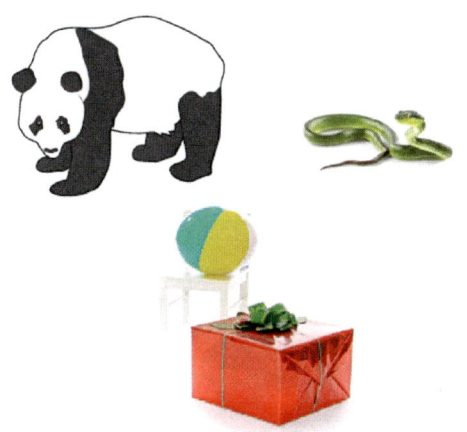

4. The ball is inside the box.

   True or False

5. The grass is shorter than the tree.

   True or False

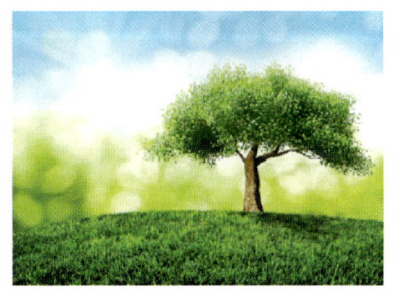

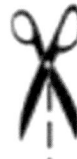

Spatial Orientation: Level 2

Instructions: For this exercise, please complete the maze starting from the top and ending at the bottom.

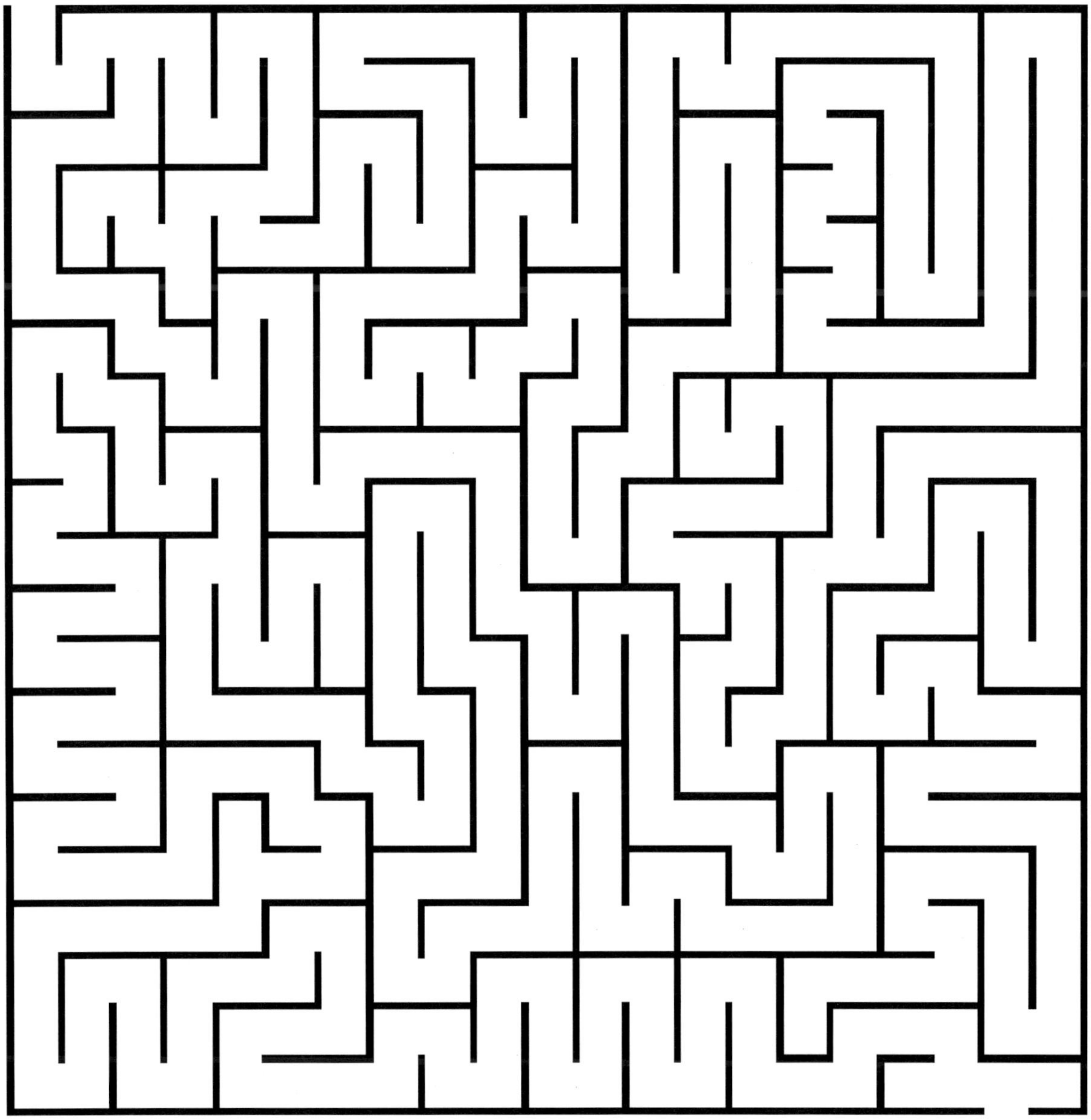

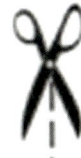

Spatial Orientation: Level 3

Instructions: For this exercise, please choose the correct word from the word box that describes the relation of the circle to the square.

Near	Below	Above
Around	Inside	To the side of

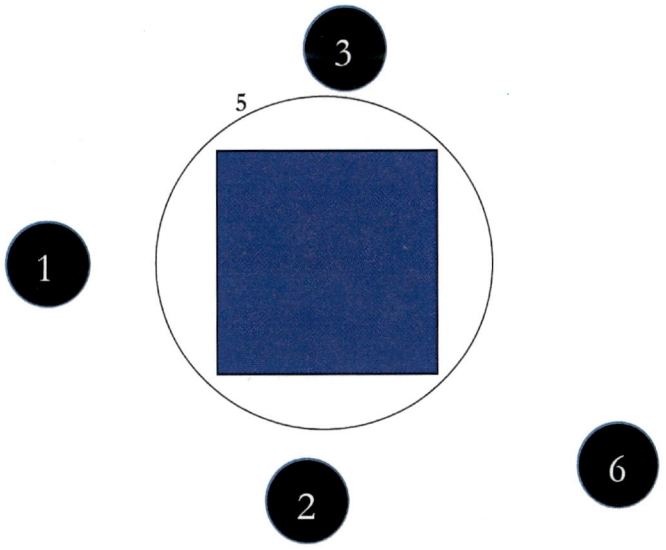

1. _____

2. _____

3. _____

4. _____

5. _____

6. _____

Answer Key

Lesson 1: Visual Recognition

Level 1: 1. dog 2. paint 3. nose 4. ladybug 5. sand 6. jaguar 7. ball 8. foot 9. monkey 10. house 11. umbrella 12. goat 13. wheel 14. cane

Level 2: 1. no 2. bee 3. bear 4. angel 5. gator 6. friend 7. left 8. pit 9. saw 10. child 11. reverse 12. diary 13. quiet 14. rain

Level 3: 1. spaghetti 2. cinnamon 3. pear 4. right 5. hare 6. a lone 7. tail 8. nun 9. time 10. mane 11. break 12. waste 13. stair 14. cereal

Lesson 2: Visual Memory

Level 1: 1. pencil 2. ball 3. hammer 4. hat 5. fan 6. book 7. clock

Level 2: 1. car 2. lamp 3. racket 4. ring 5. banana 6. acorn 7. box 8. tree 9. bear

Level 3: 1. ruler 2. eagle 3. apple 4. bicycle 5. airplane 6. canoe 7. bus 8. seesaw 9. beach 10. flower

Lesson 3: Visual Sequencing

Level 1: 1. 837564912 2. 741865932 3. 2431

Level 2: 1. 465238719 2. 65418732 3. 3421 4. CALENDAR

Level 3: 1. 4561327 2. 3562741 3. 1234 4. ROCKETSHIP; CHEMISTRY

Lesson 4: Auditory Recognition

Level 1: 1. L 2. F 3. B 4. N 5. T 6. S 7. O 8. U 9. D 10. R

Level 2: 1. TO 2. NAT 3. PUT 4. PIG 5. VAN 6. JET 7. SUN 8. RAM 9. SNAIL 10. MATCH

Level 3: 1. BALL 2. MALL 3. HIKE 4. SOAP 5. JUICE 6. BOOT 7. DRILL 8. TREE 9. PEAR 10. SHEEP

Lesson 5: Auditory Memory

Level 1: 1. A F B N M Q 2. H Y W P C D S X 3. K T E G I J L O R

Level 2: 1. Blue Apple Nine Note Phone Fan 2. Shield Box Elevator Sun Map Pencil Tape Water 3. Lock Orange Wolf Book Helmet Football Card Notebook Folder

Level 3: Have someone else rate how close the stories are from 1-10.

Lesson 6: Auditory Sequencing

Level 1: 1. SPRING 2. GRASS 3. PILLOW 4. SCHOOL 5. STATE

Level 2: 1. TELEVISION 2. CALCULATOR 3. BUILDING 4. PICTURE 5. SCIENCE

Level 3: 1. The owner treats his dog well. 2. I stopped at my friend's house. 3. The surprise party is tomorrow. 4. My charger for the computer broke. 5. We are going to see animals.

Lesson 7: Body Perception

Level 1: (From top to bottom of left side then top to bottom on right side)
1. Forehead 2. Neck 3. Right hand 4. Right knee 5. Foot 6. Left ear 7. Chest
8. Stomach 9. Thigh 10. Left leg

Level 2: (From top to bottom of left side then top to bottom on right side)
1. Monitor 2. Printer 3. Mouse 4. Power cord 5. Disk drive 6. Keyboard

Level 3: (From top to bottom of left side then top to bottom on right side)
1. Windshield wipers 2. Windshield 3. Hood 4. Front bumper 5. Headlights 6. Mirror
7. Door 8. Tire rim 9. Tire

Lesson 8: Spatial Orientation

Level 1: 1. True 2. True 3. False 4. False 5. True

Level 2: The maze should have one continuous line from the start point to the end point.

Level 3: 1. To the side of 2. Below 3. Above 4. Inside 5. Around 6. Near

Additional Resources

Overcoming Dyslexia: A New And Complete Science Based Program For Reading Problems At Any Level

By: Sally E. Shaywitz

The Dyslexia Empowerment Plan

By: Ben Foss

The Dyslexic Advantage

By: Brock Eide and Fernette Eide

The Gift of Dyslexia

By: Ronald D Davis

The Big Picture: Rethinking Dyslexia

By: Sir Richard Branson

It's Called Dyslexia

By: Jennifer Moore-Mallinos

The Elevator Project Special Needs Program

The Elevator Project Special Needs Program is committed to enabling individuals with learning disabilities to climb out of poverty by providing individualized apprenticeships programs, tailored vocational training, and a one-on-one mentor program and foster a pay it forward approach through its elevator model.

I started The Elevator Project Special Needs Program in 2014 on the notion of paying it forward or "sending the elevator down" in my community.

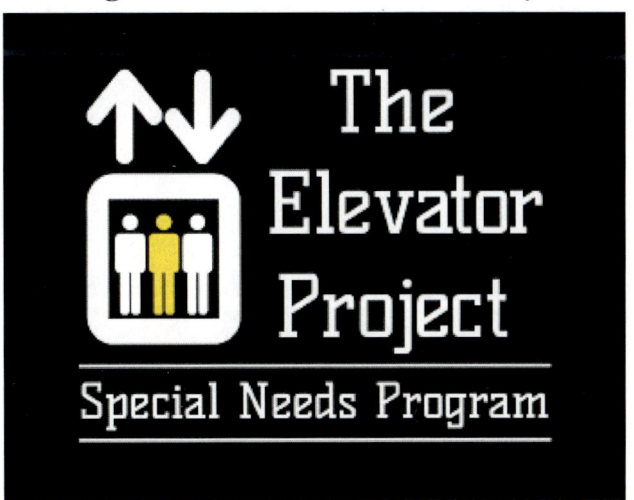

There are 6 floors in the program.

- The **Ground Floor** is the application, diagnostic, and interview process. Once participants are selected, we map out their "elevator ride".

- The **First Floor** is the in-field training level where we match an apprenticeship opportunity with our participant's interests, chosen career path, and learning

- disability.

- The **Second Floor** is the hard skills training level where participants attend customized vocational training courses in the field of their choosing for varying lengths of time.

- The **Third Floor** is the tailored soft skills training with self-identification using an EQ test, interpersonal skills, and other job readiness items such as resume writing and interview training.

- The **Fourth Floor** is where participants begin the well-waging job search and application process under our guidance.

- The final **Roof-Top Floor** is where participants have the opportunity to "send the elevator back down" for someone else to use, by serving as a mentor for a new participant in the apprenticeship floor.

This organization has helped many families rise out of poverty and will continue to do so, as we continue to grow it. For more information, visit

www.theelevatorproject.org.